The Truth About Leptin Resistance Guide

Disclaimer and Terms of Use:

Effort has been made to ensure that the information in this book is accurate and complete, however, the author and the publisher do not warrant the accuracy of the information, text and graphics contained within the book due to the rapidly changing nature of science, research, known and unknown facts and internet. The Author and the publisher do not hold any responsibility for errors, omissions or contrary interpretation of the subject matter herein. This book is presented solely for motivational and informational purposes only.

Table of Contents

Introduction

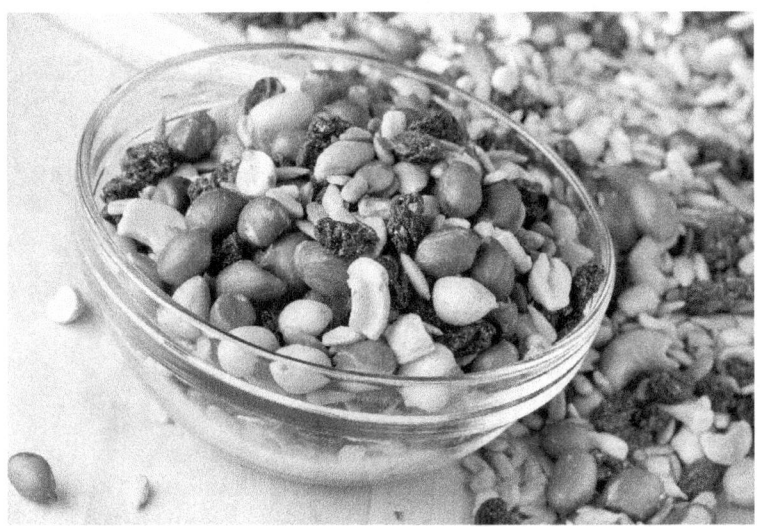

Countless individuals struggle to lose weight and, for many of them, it is a losing battle. While there are many factors which contribute to weight gain and which might interfere with your weight loss, scientists agree that one of the leading causes of obesity is related to a hormone called leptin. The leptin hormone is not what causes weight gain – it is resistance to that hormone which is one of the leading factors contributing to weight gain and difficulty with weight loss. If you are struggling to lose weight, you would do well to learn the basics about leptin and leptin resistance to see if it might be affecting you. In this book, you will learn what leptin is, how it affects your body, and how it might be contributing to your difficulties with weight loss. You will also receive tips for overcoming leptin resistance as well as an assortment of healthy recipes to support your weight loss efforts.

What is Leptin?

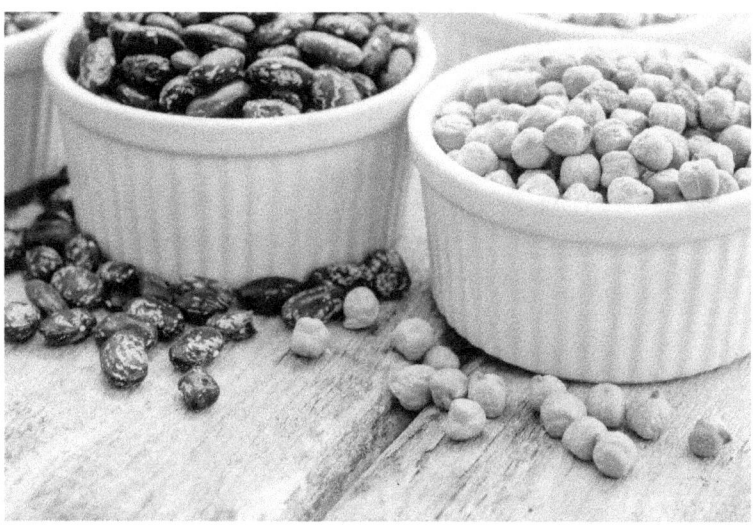

Leptin is a type of hormone that plays an important role in regulating your energy intake and your energy expenditure. In short, it is the hormone that sends signals to your brain to tell you that you are hungry – it is also the hormone that tells your brain when you have eaten enough. Insulin is another type of hormone and it works closely with leptin to produce these effects in the body. Leptin is produced by your fat cells and, in addition to telling your brain to stop eating when you are full, it also stops your body from storing fat and signals for it to begin burning off some of the extra fat that has been stored. When your body doesn't respond appropriately to leptin levels in your blood, it can lead to weight gain and obesity.

What is Leptin Resistance?

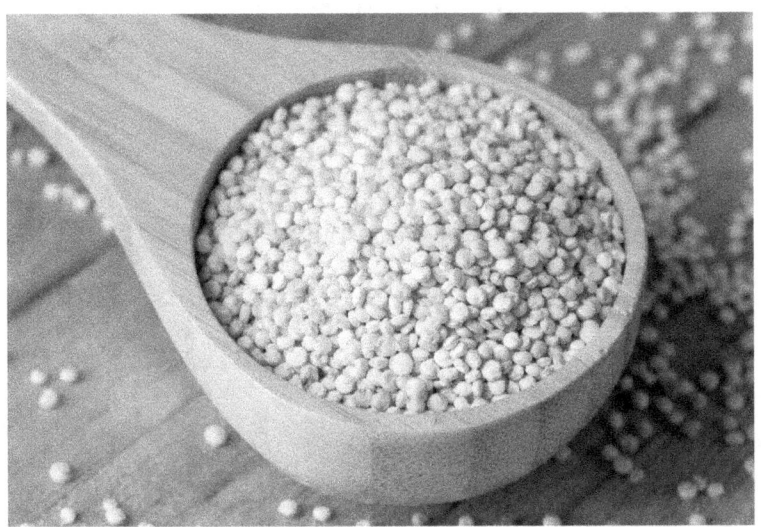

Leptin resistance is a condition in which the body stops responding appropriately to leptin levels in the blood. When your energy stores get low, your fat cells start to produce leptin which signals your brain and tells you that you are hungry. As a result, you eat until your fat stores have been replenished and then your body sends a signal to your brain telling you that you are full and you should stop eating. If you follow a diet that is high in sugar, grains, and processed foods, you may experience chronic inflammation which could impair your body's ability to read and respond to leptin levels. By eating a lot of sugars and processed grains, your body will also continuously produce high levels of leptin and, eventually, your body will develop a resistance to it. When your body becomes resistant to leptin you do not get that signal telling you that you are full and you should stop eating. As a result, you eat more than you really need to and a lot of the excess calories will be stored as fat.

How to Combat Leptin Resistance

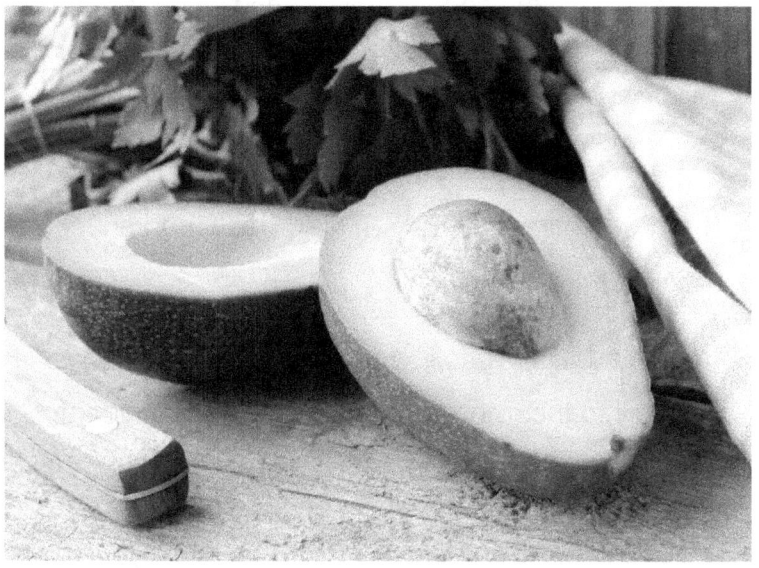

Diet and exercise are the keys to combating leptin resistance. When you follow a diet high in sugars, grains, and processed foods, your blood sugar levels will be very high and that contributes to leptin resistance. The key to repairing this problem, then, is to change your diet – focus on wholesome nutritious foods instead. The best diet for leptin resistance is one that is low in sugar and grains but high in healthy fats with a moderate amount of protein. In fact, a diet that consists of 50% to 70% fats is ideal for combating leptin resistance, particularly when those fats come from healthy sources like avocado, olive oil, coconut oil, grass-fed butter, and nuts. Try to eat a protein-rich breakfast and limit your carbohydrate intake throughout the day. You should also try to avoid eating very large meals, focusing instead of having several smaller meals and snacks throughout the day.

In addition to following a healthy diet, you should try to incorporate some regular exercise into your weekly routine. Nutritionist often agree that 80% of the benefits you gain from following a healthy lifestyle come from a healthy diet – the other 20% comes from exercise. You do not necessarily need to become a marathon runner to combat leptin resistance, but you should aim for 20 to 30 minutes of moderate exercise about 3 to 5 times a week. This might be as simple as taking a walk, going for a quick jog, or riding your bike. It doesn't matter so much what type of exercise you do, as long as you do it regularly.

Leptin Resistance Diet Recipes

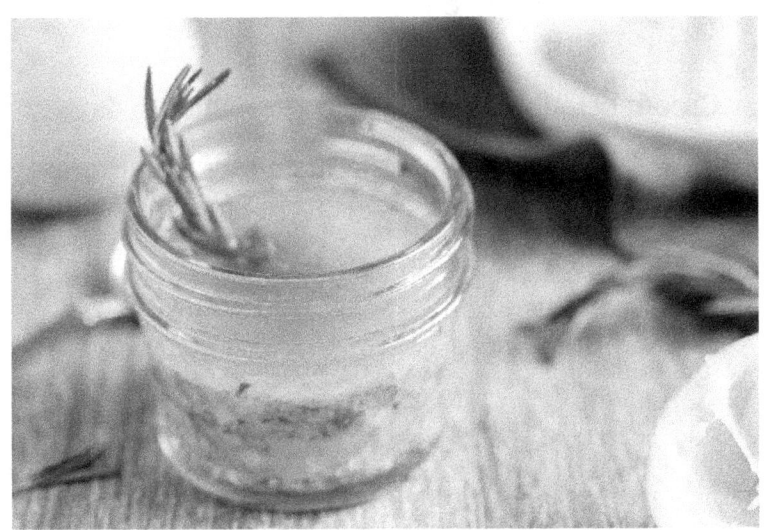

Recipes Included in this Book:

Raspberry Overnight Oats

Avocado, Spinach and Lime Smoothie

Zucchini and Red Pepper Frittata

Banana Protein Pancakes

Lemon, Zucchini and Kiwi Smoothie

Eggs Baked in Red Peppers

Tomato Omelet with Fresh Basil

Roasted Butternut Squash Soup

Cucumber, Red Onion and Dill Salad

Ginger Carrot Sweet Potato Soup

Curried Egg Salad on Lettuce

Cream of Cauliflower Soup

Spinach Salad with Avocado and Almonds

Cream of Mushroom Soup

Tomato Mozzarella Salad

Chocolate Chia Protein Smoothie

Kiwi Banana Protein Shake

Cucumber Mint Protein Smoothie

Raspberry Overnight Oats

Servings: 2

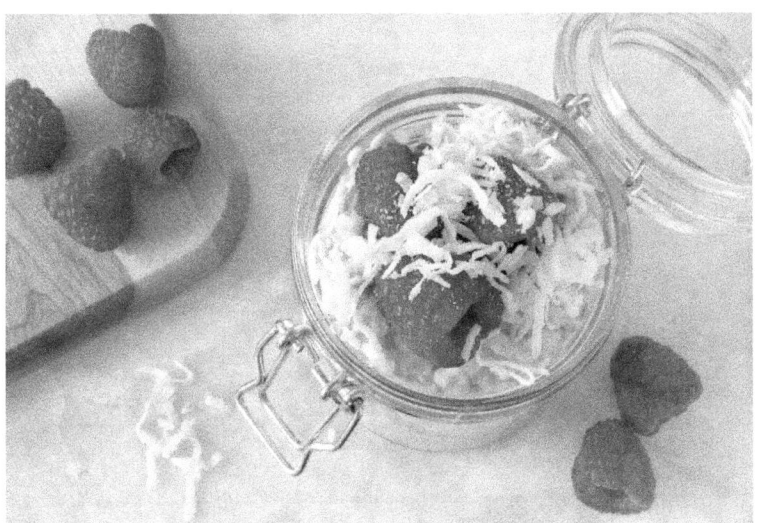

Ingredients:

¾ cups old-fashioned oats, uncooked

½ cup skim milk or almond milk

1 tablespoon raw honey

1 teaspoon vanilla extract

Pinch salt

Instructions:

1. Combine all of the ingredients in a bowl and stir well.
2. Cover and chill overnight.

3. Spoon the oatmeal into bowls and serve with raspberries and shredded coconut.

Avocado, Spinach and Lime Smoothie

Servings: 1 to 2

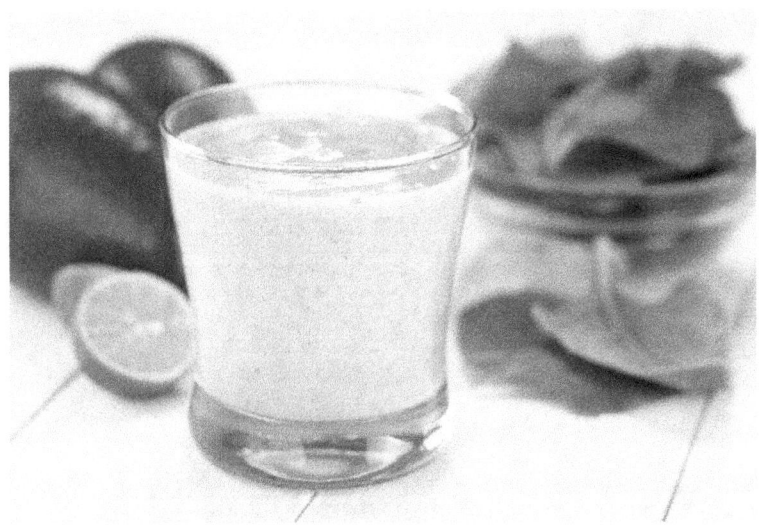

Ingredients:

1 ½ cups fresh chopped spinach

½ ripe avocado, pitted and chopped

1 cup water

½ cup plain Greek yogurt

2 tablespoons fresh lime juice

Instructions:

1. Combine all of the ingredients in a high-speed blender.
2. Blend on high speed for 30 to 60 seconds until smooth and well combined.

3. Pour into two smoothie glasses and enjoy
    immediately.

Zucchini and Red Pepper Frittata

Servings: 6

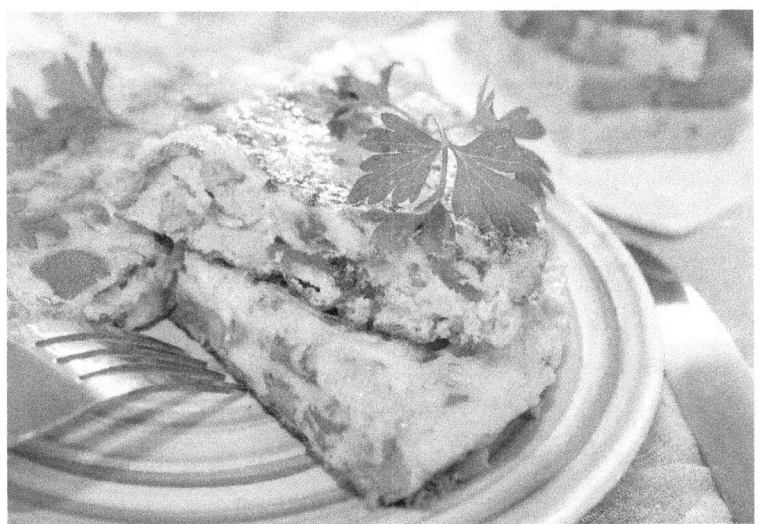

Ingredients:

1 tablespoon coconut oil

1 small zucchini, peeled and diced

1 medium red pepper, cored and diced

½ cup diced yellow onion

8 large eggs, beaten

3 to 4 tablespoons water

Salt and pepper to taste

½ cup shredded cheddar cheese

Instructions:

1. Preheat your broiler to high heat while you prepare the frittata.
2. Melt the coconut oil in an oven-proof skillet over medium heat.
3. Stir in the zucchini, red pepper and onion then cook for 5 to 6 minutes until tender.
4. Whisk together the eggs, water, salt and pepper.
5. Pour the eggs into the skillet and stir gently – cook for 3 to 4 minutes until the egg is almost set.
6. Sprinkle with shredded cheese and place under the broiler for 2 minutes or until the egg is set and the cheese is melted.
7. Let the frittata rest for 5 minutes before serving.

Banana Protein Pancakes

Servings: 4

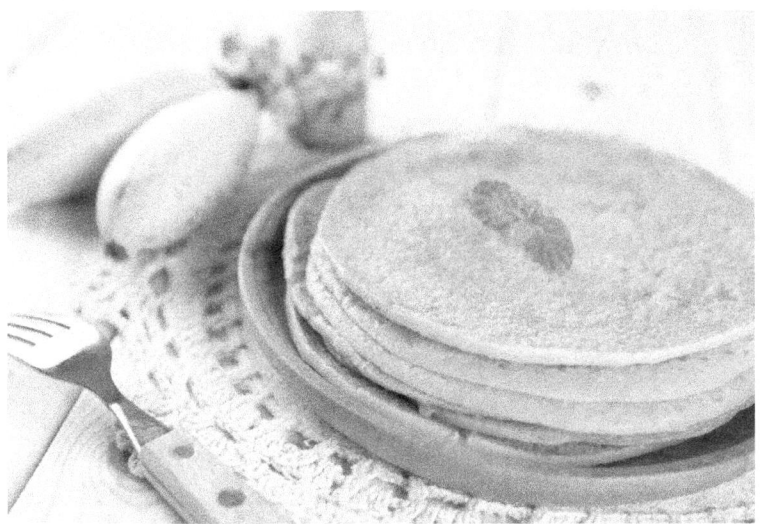

Ingredients:

3 medium overripe bananas, mashed

2 large eggs plus 1 egg white, whisked

½ cup plus 1 tablespoon vanilla protein powder

½ teaspoon ground cinnamon

Instructions:

1. Combine the banana, eggs, protein powder and cinnamon in a food processor.
2. Blend until smooth and well combined.
3. Heat a large nonstick skillet over medium heat and grease with oil.

4. Spoon the batter into the skillet, using about 2 to 3 tablespoons per pancake.
5. Cook for 2 to 3 minutes until the underside is browned then flip and cook until the other side is browned.

Lemon, Zucchini and Kiwi Smoothie

Servings: 1 to 2

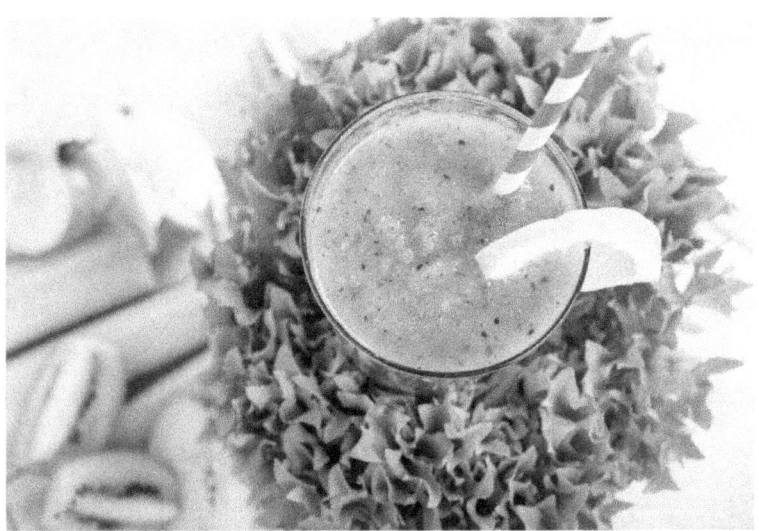

Ingredients:

2 ripe kiwi fruit, peeled and sliced

1 small zucchini, peeled and chopped

1 small, frozen banana, peeled and sliced

1 cup water

2 tablespoons fresh lemon juice

Instructions:

1. Combine all of the ingredients in a high-speed blender.
2. Blend on high speed for 30 to 60 seconds until smooth and well combined.

3. Pour into two smoothie glasses and enjoy immediately.

Eggs Baked in Red Peppers

Servings: 4

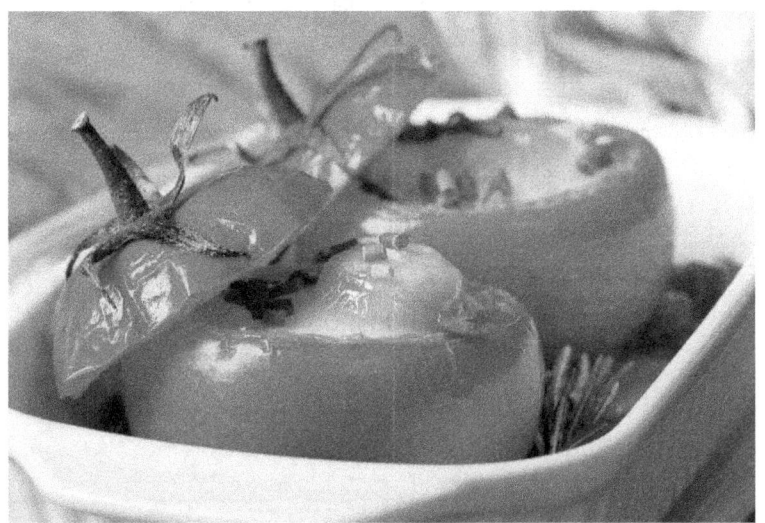

Ingredients:

4 large red bell peppers

1 cup frozen spinach, thawed

¼ cup diced yellow onion

¼ cup shredded cheddar cheese

2 tablespoons fresh chopped chives

4 large eggs

Salt and pepper to taste

Instructions:

1. Preheat the oven to 400°F (205°C).

2. Cut the tops off the red peppers and scoop out the seeds and membrane.
3. Place the peppers upright in a square glass baking dish.
4. Squeeze the water out of the spinach and stir it together with the cheese, onions and chives.
5. Spoon the spinach mixture into the peppers and crack an egg into each.
6. Sprinkle with salt and pepper to taste then bake for 15 to 20 minutes until the egg is set.

Tomato Omelet with Fresh Basil

Servings: 1

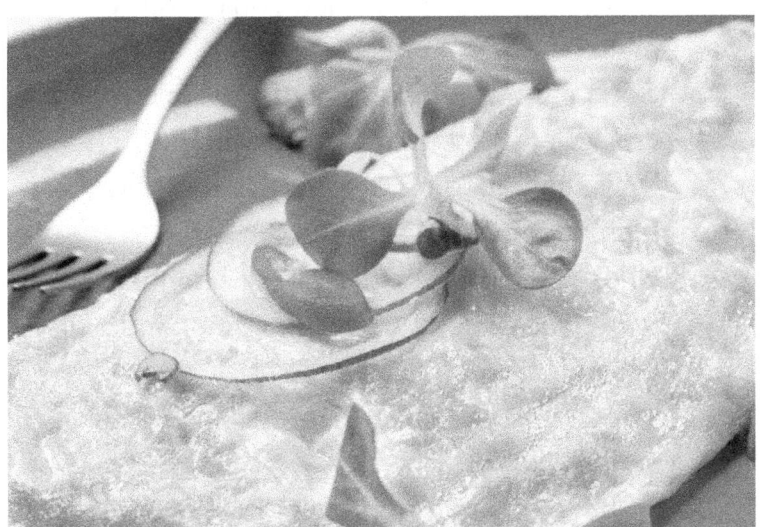

Ingredients:

2 teaspoons coconut oil

1 medium ripe tomato, chopped

3 tablespoons minced onion

1 clove minced garlic

2 large eggs

1 tablespoon water

1 tablespoon chopped chives

Instructions:

1. Heat 1 teaspoon oil in a small skillet over medium heat.
2. Add the tomato, onion and garlic – cook for 3 minutes, stirring often.
3. Spoon the vegetables into a bowl and reheat the skillet with the rest of the oil.
4. Whisk together the eggs, water and chives then pour into the skillet.
5. Cook for 2 minutes then tilt the pan to spread the uncooked egg – cook another minute or two until the egg is almost set.
6. Spoon the vegetables over half the omelet and sprinkle with basil.
7. Fold the empty half of the omelet over the filling and cook for 30 to 60 seconds until the egg is set.

Roasted Butternut Squash Soup

Servings: 6 to 8

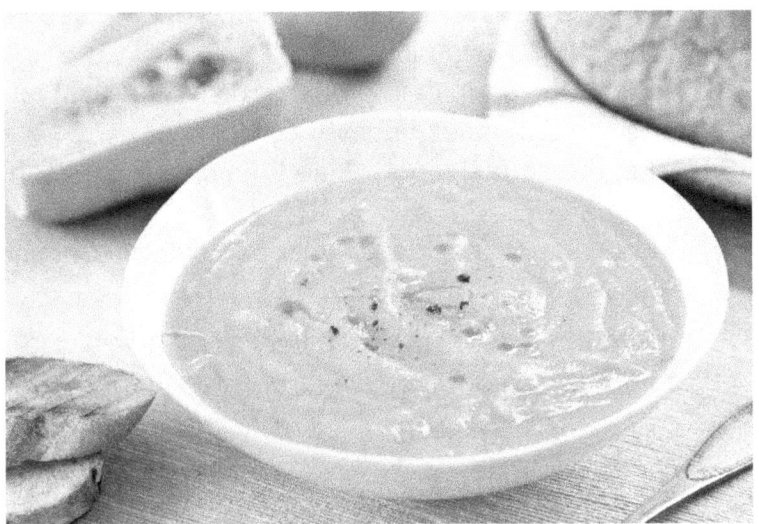

Ingredients:

2 large butternut squash

2 tablespoons coconut oil

1 large yellow onion, chopped

2 small carrots, peeled and chopped

1 large stalk celery, sliced

1 tablespoon minced garlic

5 ½ cups chicken or vegetable broth

1 teaspoon fresh chopped thyme

Salt and pepper to taste

Instructions:

1. Preheat the oven to 350°F (180°C).
2. Cut the squash in half and scoop out the seeds then brush with oil.
3. Place the squash in a baking dish and roast for 35 to 45 minutes until very tender.
4. Let the squash cool a little then scoop the flesh into a bowl.
5. Heat the oil in a large saucepan over medium heat.
6. Add the onion, carrots, celery and garlic – cook for 6 to 8 minutes until tender.
7. Stir in the remaining ingredients (including the squash) then bring to a boil.
8. Reduce heat and simmer on low for 20 to 25 minutes until the vegetables are very tender.
9. Remove from heat and puree the soup using an immersion blender.
10. Season with salt and pepper to taste – serve hot.

Cucumber, Red Onion and Dill Salad

Servings: 6

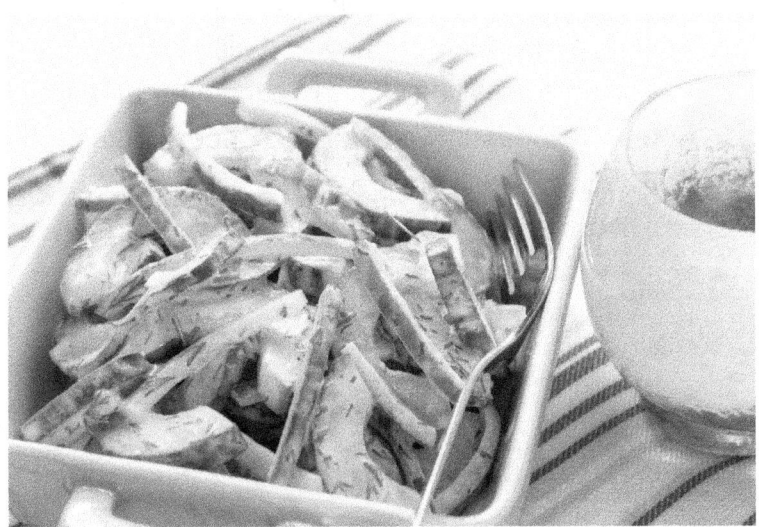

Ingredients:

2 large seedless cucumbers, sliced thin

1 medium red onion, sliced thin

¼ cup canned coconut milk

3 tablespoons rice vinegar

2 tablespoons fresh chopped dill

1 tablespoon raw honey

Salt and pepper to taste

Instructions:

1. Combine the cucumber and red onion in a bowl.
2. In a separate bowl, whisk together the coconut milk, rice vinegar, honey and dill.
3. Toss the dressing with the cucumber and red onion – season with salt and pepper to taste.
4. Cover and chill until ready to serve.

Ginger Carrot Sweet Potato Soup

Servings: 6

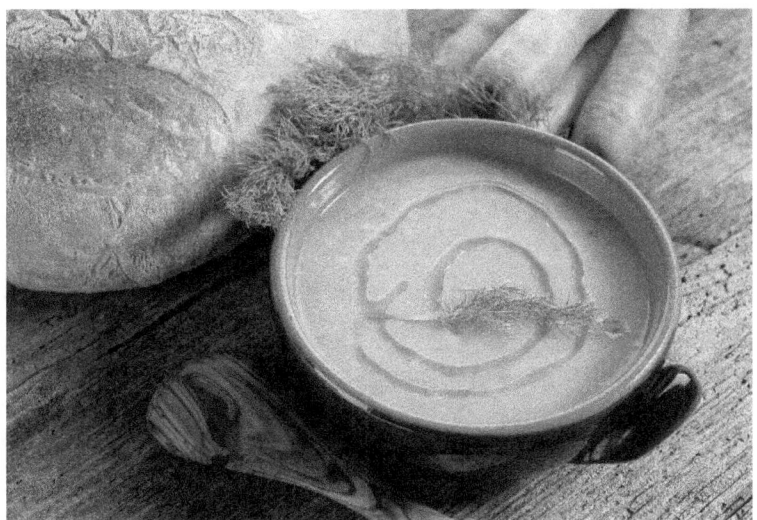

Ingredients:

1 tablespoon coconut oil

1 large yellow onion, chopped

1 lbs. fresh sliced carrots

1 large sweet potato, peeled and chopped

1 tablespoon fresh grated ginger

4 cups chicken or vegetable broth

1 cup water

1 tablespoon fresh lemon juice

Salt and pepper to taste

Instructions:

1. Heat the oil in a large saucepan over medium heat.
2. Add the onion, carrots, sweet potato and ginger – cook for 6 to 8 minutes until tender.
3. Stir in the remaining ingredients then bring to a boil.
4. Reduce heat and simmer on low for 20 to 25 minutes until the vegetables are very tender.
5. Remove from heat and puree the soup using an immersion blender.
6. Season with salt and pepper to taste – serve hot.

Curried Egg Salad on Lettuce

Servings: 6

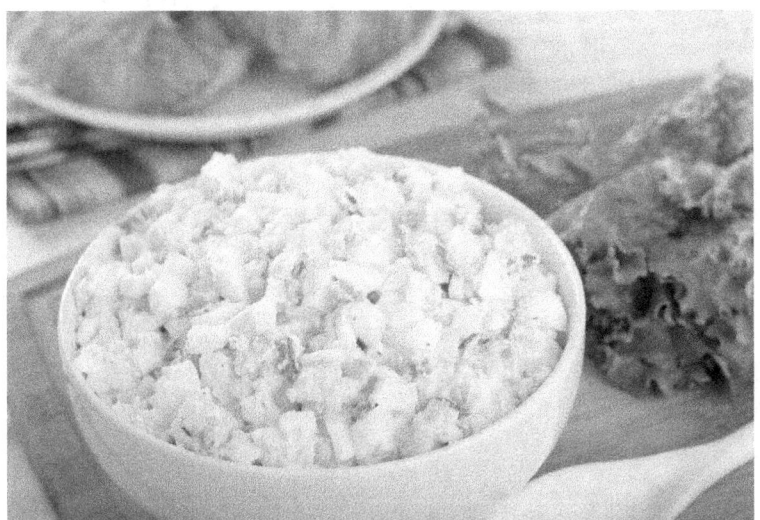

Ingredients:

1 large ripe avocado, pitted and chopped

2 tablespoons mayonnaise

1 teaspoon curry powder

1 teaspoon Dijon mustard

10 large hardboiled eggs, peeled and chopped

¼ cup diced red onion

1 stalk celery, diced

Salt and pepper to taste

Instructions:

1. Mash the avocado in a bowl with the mayonnaise, curry powder, and mustard.
2. Fold in the chopped eggs, red onion and celery – season with salt and pepper to taste.
3. Chill for at least an hour then serve over a bed of lettuce.

Cream of Cauliflower Soup

Servings: 6 to 8

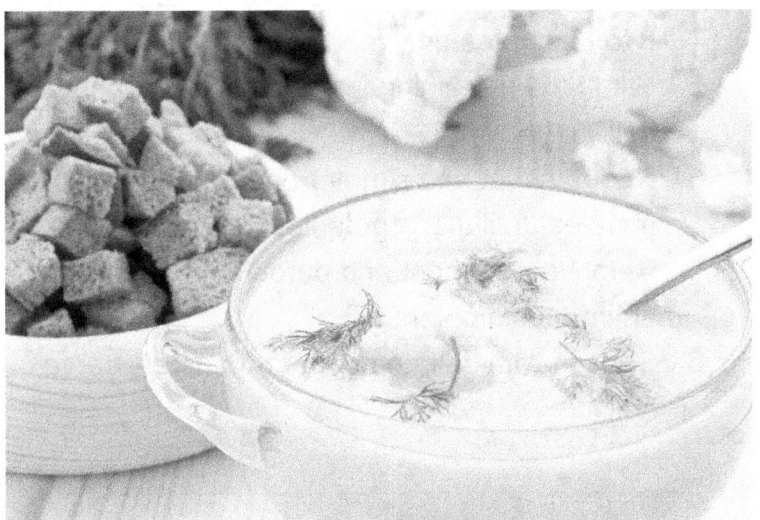

Ingredients:

2 tablespoons coconut oil

1 large yellow onion, chopped

9 cups fresh chopped cauliflower

1 ½ tablespoons minced garlic

5 cups chicken broth or vegetable broth

1 cup canned coconut milk

Salt and pepper to taste

Instructions:

1. Heat the oil in a large saucepan over medium heat.
2. Add the onion, cauliflower and garlic – cook for 6 to 8 minutes until tender.
3. Stir in the remaining ingredients then bring to a boil.
4. Reduce heat and simmer on low for 20 to 25 minutes until the vegetables are very tender.
5. Remove from heat and puree the soup using an immersion blender.
6. Season with salt and pepper to taste – serve hot.

Spinach Salad with Avocado and Almonds

Servings: 4

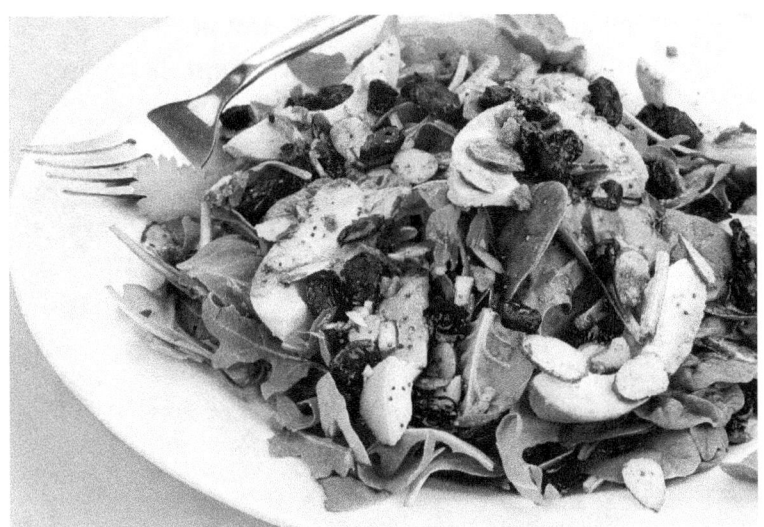

Ingredients:

6 cups fresh baby spinach, packed

1 medium ripe avocado, pitted and sliced thin

½ cup seedless raisins

¼ cup thinly sliced almonds

¼ cup olive oil

2 tablespoons balsamic vinegar

1 teaspoon red wine vinegar

1 teaspoon raw honey

Pinch salt and pepper

Instructions:

1. Toss the spinach, avocado, almonds and raisins together in a large salad bowl.
2. Whisk together the remaining ingredients in a separate bowl.
3. Serve the salad drizzled with the dressing.

Cream of Mushroom Soup

Servings: 6

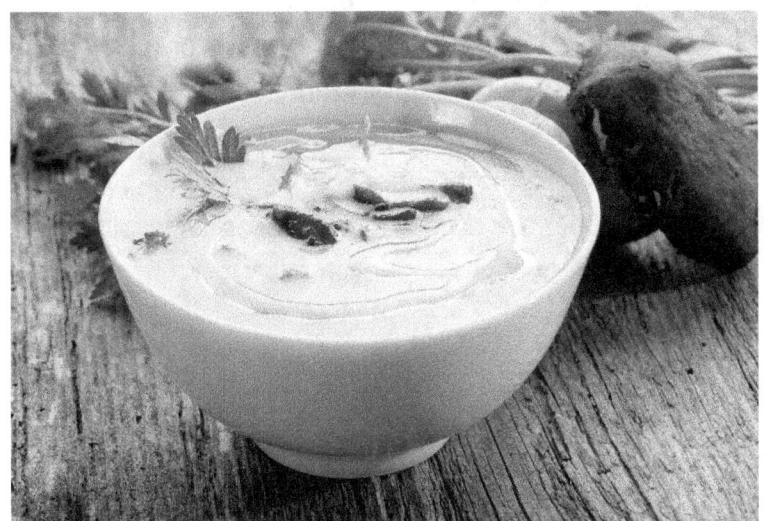

Ingredients:

2 tablespoons coconut oil

1 medium yellow onion, chopped

2 ½ lbs. sliced mushrooms

5 cups vegetable broth

¾ cups heavy cream

Salt and pepper to taste

Instructions:

1. Heat the oil in a large saucepan over medium heat.

2. Add the onion, mushrooms and garlic – cook for 6 to 8 minutes until tender.
3. Stir in the broth then bring to a boil.
4. Reduce heat and simmer on low for 20 to 25 minutes until the vegetables are very tender.
5. Remove from heat and puree the soup using an immersion blender.
6. Whisk in the cream then season with salt and pepper to taste – serve hot.

Tomato Mozzarella Salad

Servings: 6

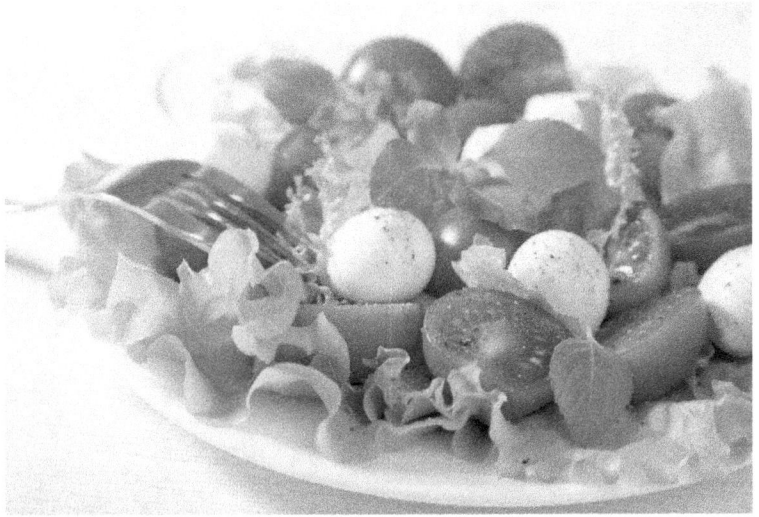

Ingredients:

2 cups cherry tomatoes, halved

½ lbs. fresh mozzarella, chopped into cubes

½ cup fresh basil leaves, coarsely chopped

2 ½ tablespoons olive oil

1 ½ tablespoons balsamic vinegar

Salt and pepper to taste

Instructions:

1. Combine the tomatoes, mozzarella, and lettuce in a salad bowl.
2. Toss with the basil, olive oil and vinegar.

3. Season with salt and pepper to taste and chill until ready to serve.

Chocolate Chia Protein Smoothie

Servings: 1 to 2

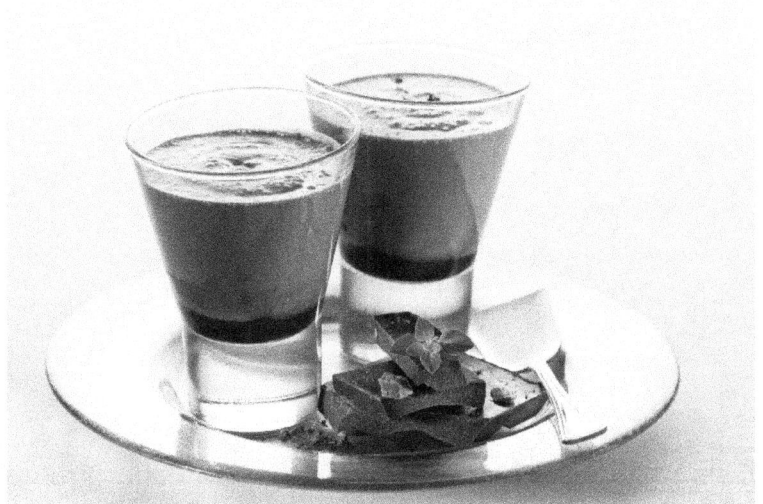

Ingredients:

1 ½ cups 2% or skim milk

1 cup ice cubes

2 scoops chocolate protein powder

3 tablespoons chia seeds

1 tablespoon raw honey

Pinch ground cinnamon

Instructions:

1. Combine all of the ingredients in a high-speed blender.

2. Blend on high speed for 30 to 60 seconds until smooth and well combined.
3. Pour into two smoothie glasses and enjoy immediately.

Kiwi Banana Protein Shake

Servings: 1 to 2

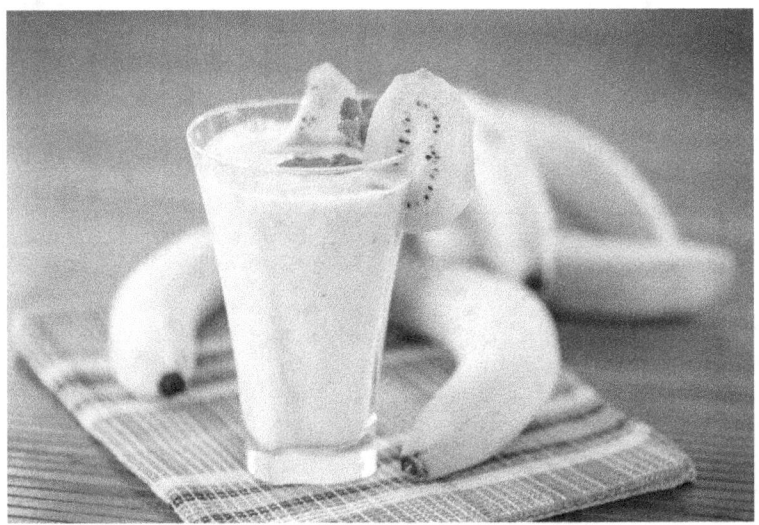

Ingredients:

1 large frozen banana, peeled and sliced

1 ripe kiwi fruit, peeled and sliced

1 cup plain Greek yogurt

½ cup ice cubes

1 scoop vanilla protein powder

Instructions:

1. Combine all of the ingredients in a high-speed blender.
2. Blend on high speed for 30 to 60 seconds until smooth and well combined.

3. Pour into two smoothie glasses and enjoy immediately.

Cucumber Mint Protein Smoothie

Servings: 1 to 2

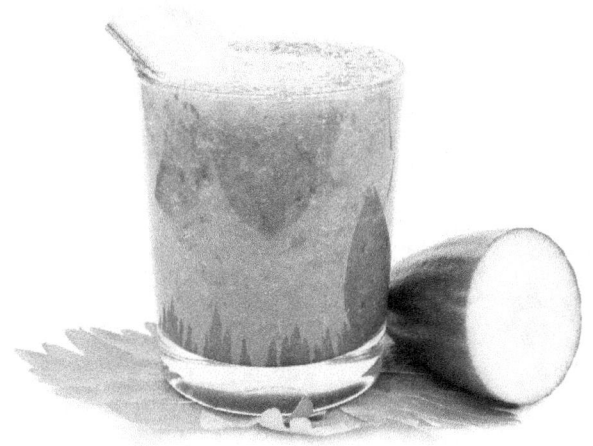

Ingredients:

1 ½ cups diced cucumber

1 ½ cups water

½ cup ice cubes

2 scoops unflavored protein powder

¼ cup fresh chopped mint

1 teaspoon raw honey

Instructions:

1. Combine all of the ingredients in a high-speed blender.

2. Blend on high speed for 30 to 60 seconds until smooth and well combined.
3. Pour into two smoothie glasses and enjoy immediately.

Conclusion

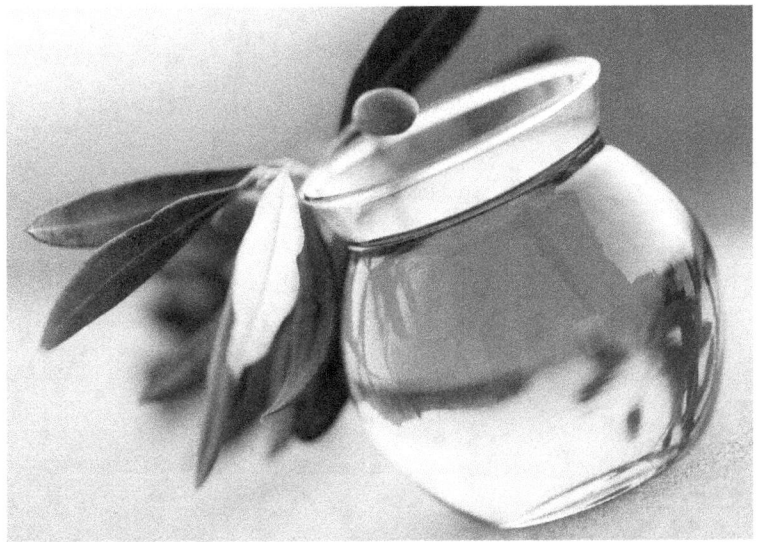

Hopefully, after reading this book, you have a better understanding of what leptin resistance is and how it might be impacting your weight loss struggles. Leptin is a very important hormone in the body and, if you do not follow a healthy diet, your body's reaction to it could become impaired and it could lead to weight gain. To combat leptin resistance you should make healthy changes to your diet and try to incorporate some exercise into your routine. If you are ready to make these changes, this book is the perfect place to start – just pick a recipe and give it a try!